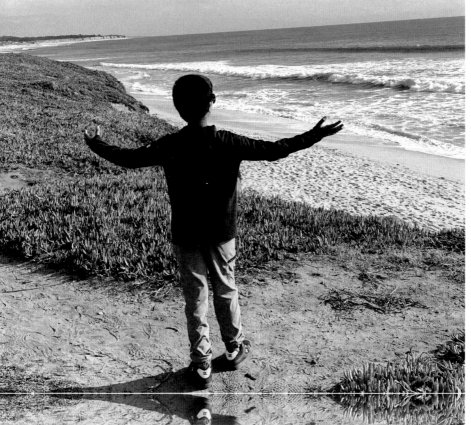

Namaskar School of Yoga & Mindfulness

NAMASTE
EARTH

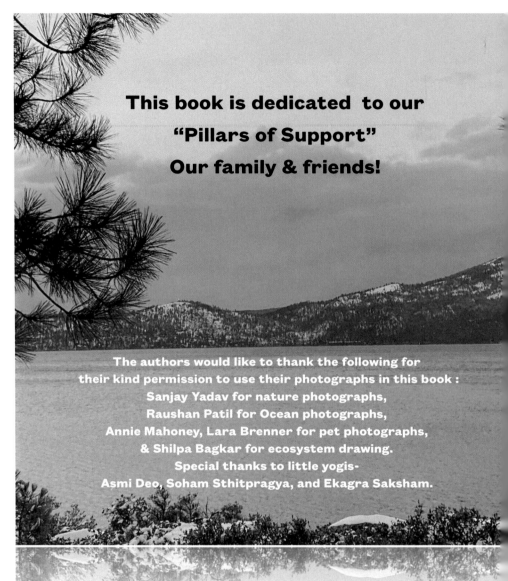

This book is dedicated to our
"Pillars of Support"
Our family & friends!

The authors would like to thank the following for
their kind permission to use their photographs in this book :
Sanjay Yadav for nature photographs,
Raushan Patil for Ocean photographs,
Annie Mahoney, Lara Brenner for pet photographs,
& Shilpa Bagkar for ecosystem drawing.
Special thanks to little yogis-
Asmi Deo, Soham Sthitpragya, and Ekagra Saksham.

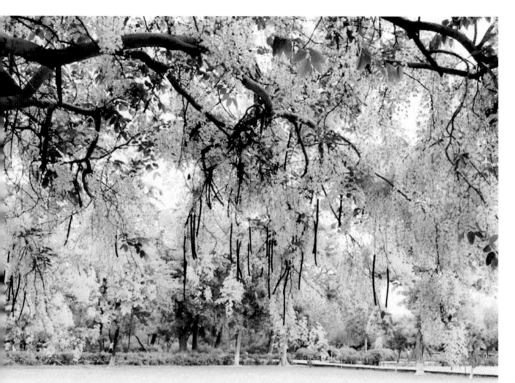

Yoga Friends,

Did you know that yoga was invented a long time ago by people who were very curious about nature? Many of the original yoga poses like Sun Salutations, Downward Facing Dog, Lotus and Tree Pose were inspired by observations of the sun rising and setting, the constellations, phases of the moon, animals, flowers and trees.

Yoga reminds us that we are all part of nature, and teaches us to take care of our health and the health of our planet, to be kind to all forms of life, to use natural resources wisely and to be thankful for the fresh air, clean water and natural beauty that surrounds and supports us. Yoga and our Earth go hand in hand! We hope this book awakens your deep-rooted connection to Mother Nature.

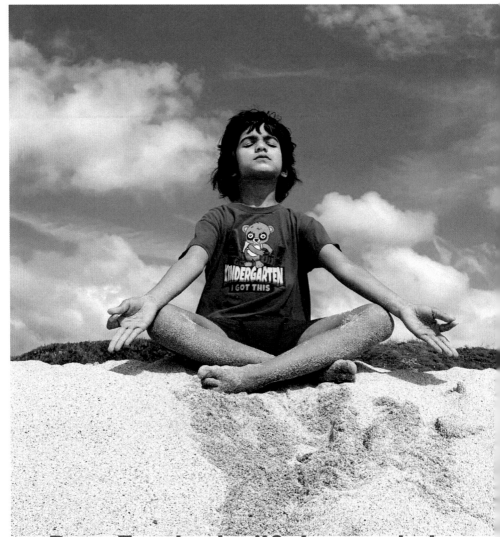

Dear Earth, the life in me admires the life in you and says, Namaste! As I sit straight, tall and mindful in your lap, I feel safe and protected, joyful and connected just the way I feel during my yoga practice.

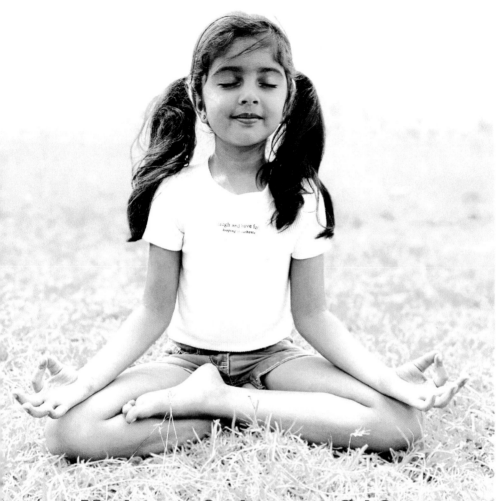

My heart feels grateful for everything you provide to make my life beautiful. Today and every day, I want to thank you and everything that belongs to you by doing yoga poses in your honor.

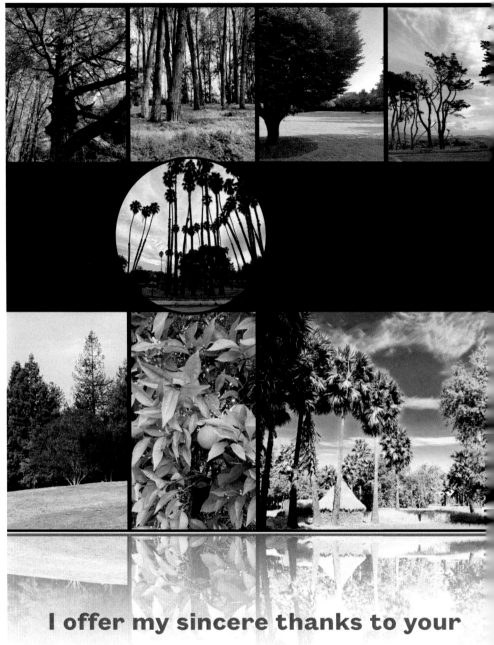

I offer my sincere thanks to your life-giving trees.

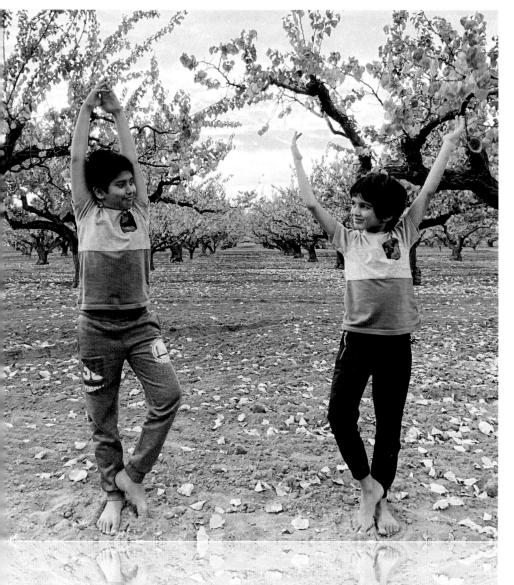

Standing in Tree Pose, as I make my roots stronger, I hold the balance, focus, and capability to be the oxygen of my world.

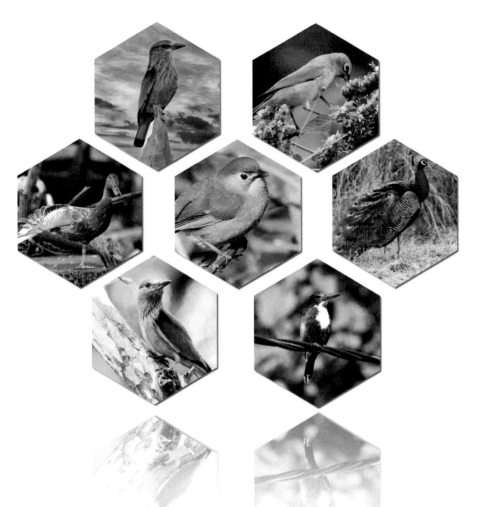

I am grateful for your birds, who
have helped shape plant life all
around the world.

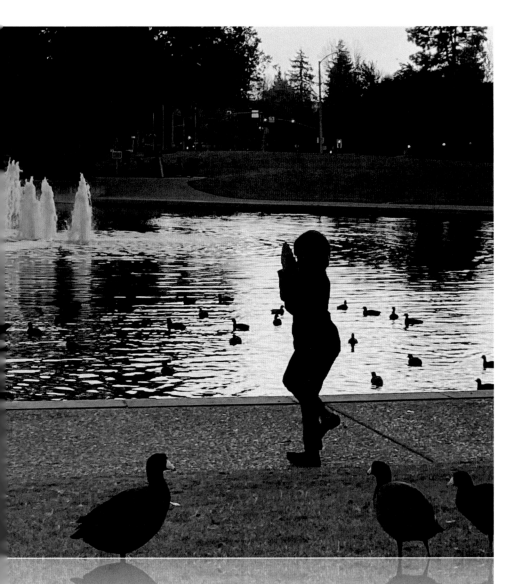

As I practice Eagle Pose, I know I will be able to fly high one day. I will see problems like climate change and pollution with my eagle eyes, and I will solve them with my inner strength.

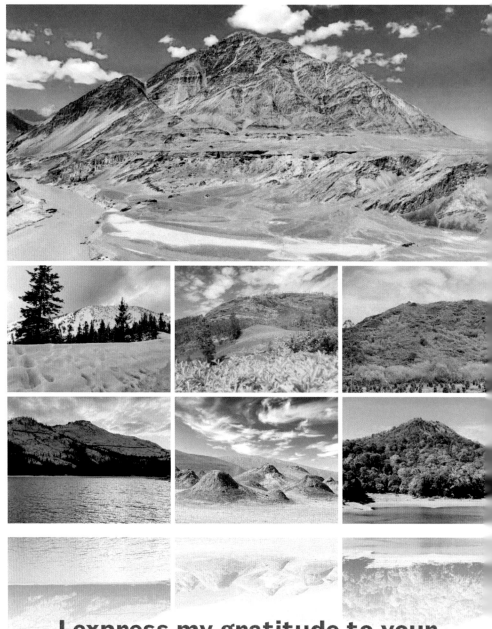

I express my gratitude to your majestic mountains.

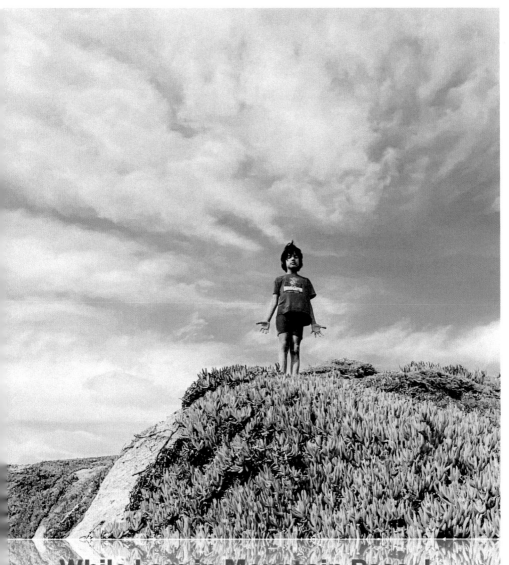

While I am in Mountain Pose, I feel the stability inside me, and I am confident that nothing can move me from my mission to bring more stability to the world.

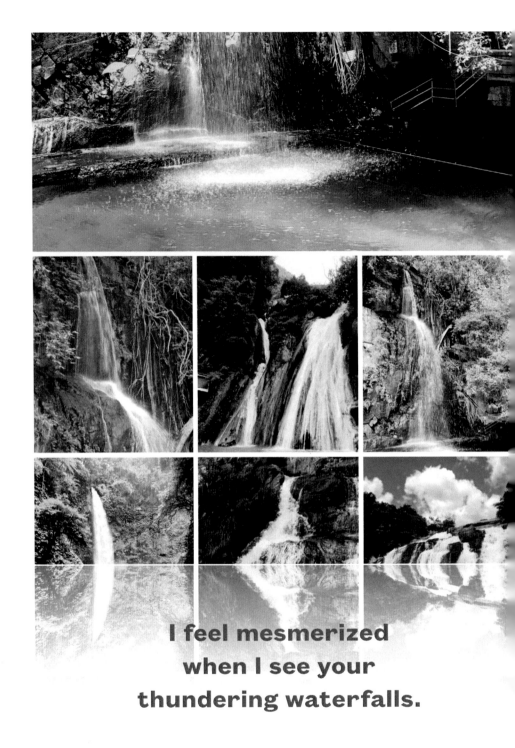

I feel mesmerized
when I see your
thundering waterfalls.

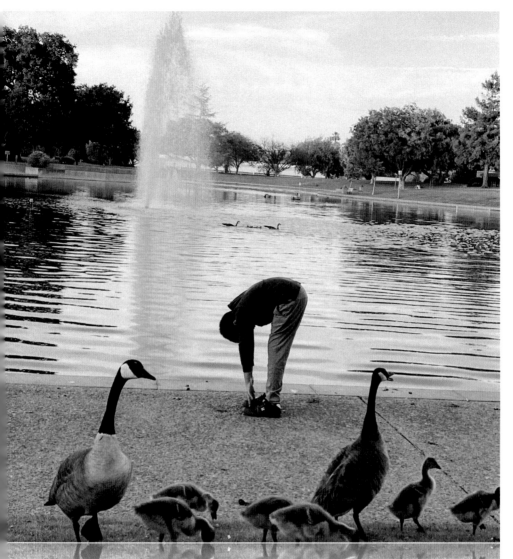

As I do Waterfall Pose, my mind is calm and invites brave and bold thoughts about new ways to support sustainability on earth.

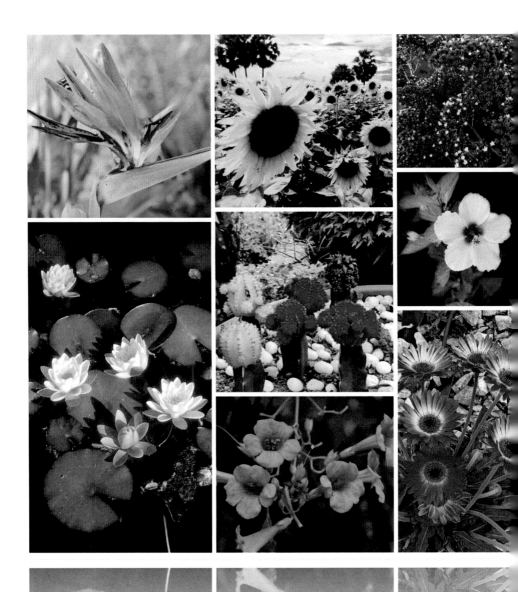

Thanks to the infinite beauty your
colorful and fragrant flowers
display all around us.

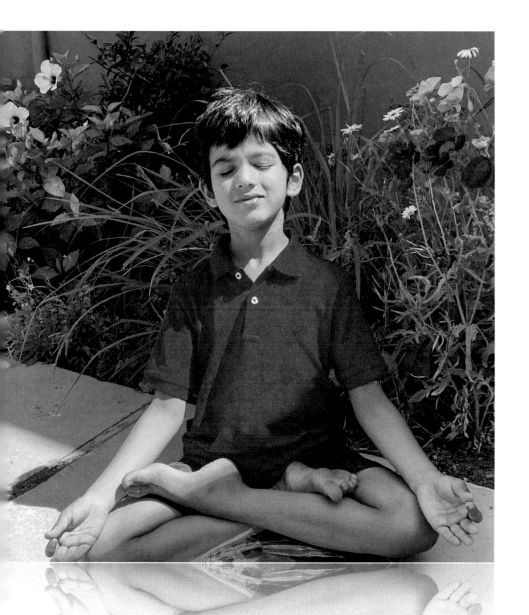

Sitting in Lotus Pose, I attain the knowledge and wisdom to ensure Planet Earth's beauty and purity.

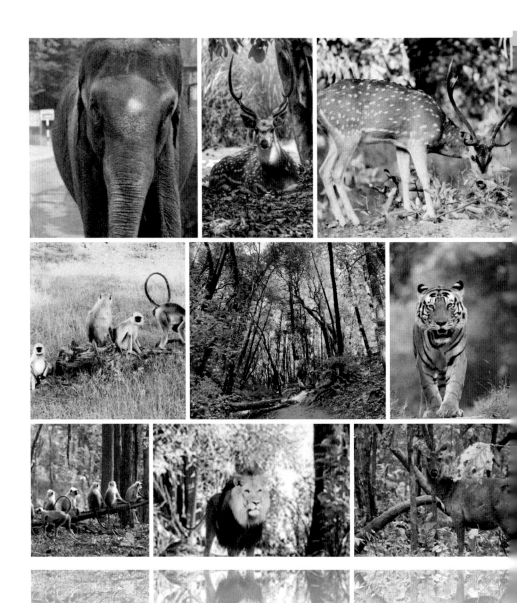

I acknowledge your forests,
the real heroes keeping the
planet healthy and alive.

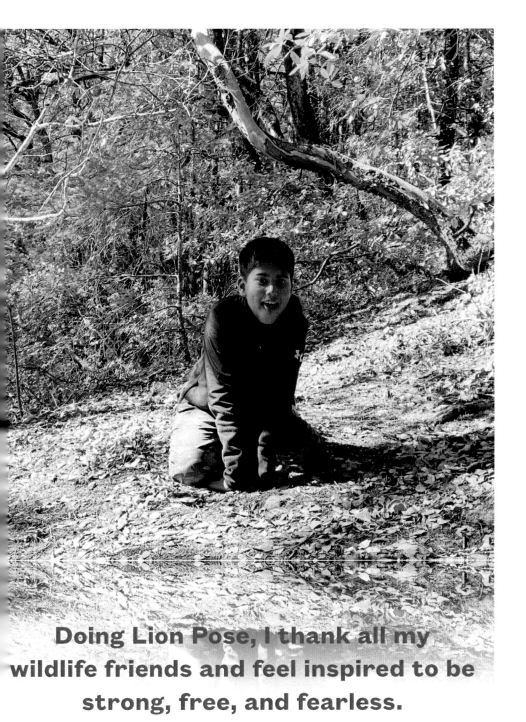

Doing Lion Pose, I thank all my
wildlife friends and feel inspired to be
strong, free, and fearless.

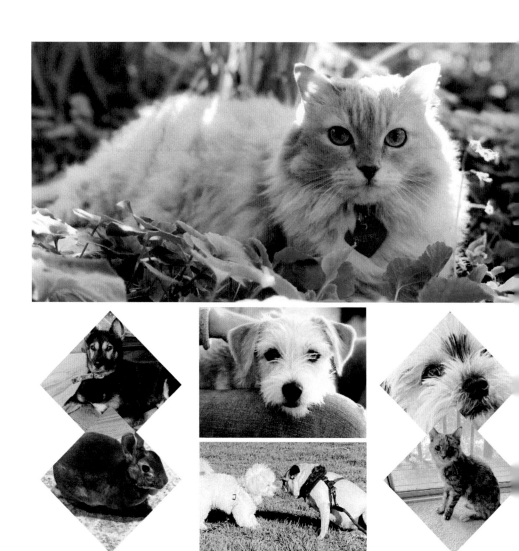

I appreciate the pets you have
given to us as friends who
teach us about trust
and unconditional love.

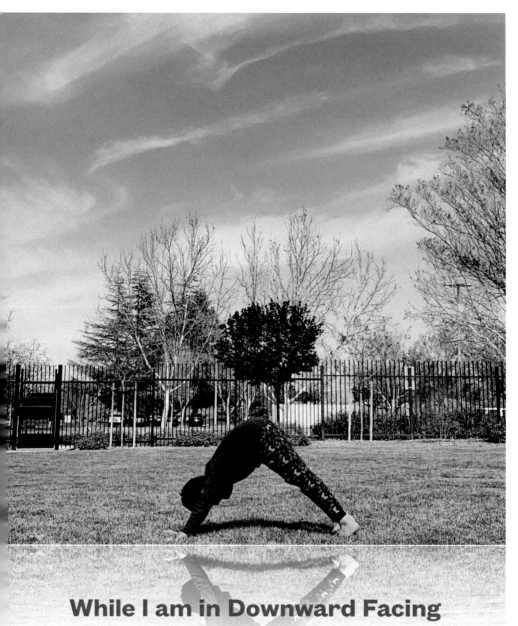

While I am in Downward Facing Dog Pose, I become aware of a strong bond between me and everything around me.

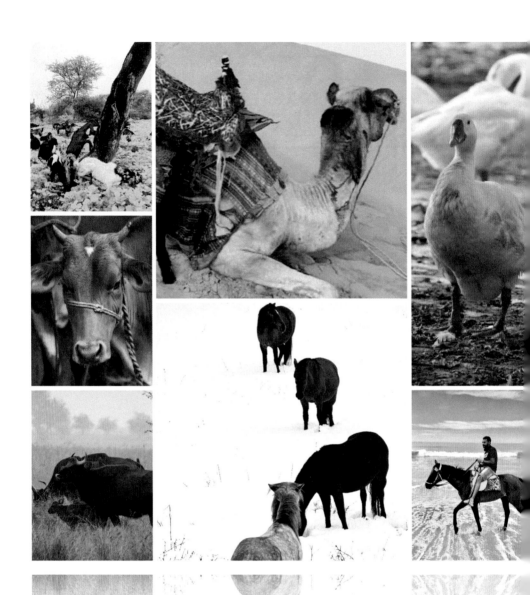

How can I forget to say thanks
to all of the farm animals who
have long been the backbone
of human civilization?

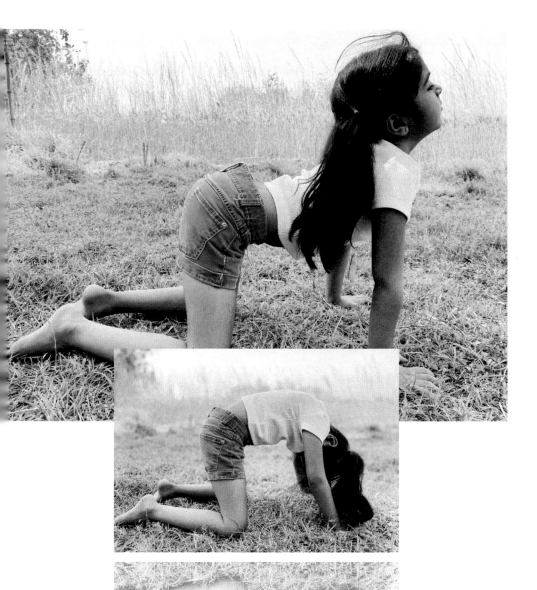

Cat and Cow Pose reminds me
that just as I need to take care of
my spine, I also need to protect
the environment.

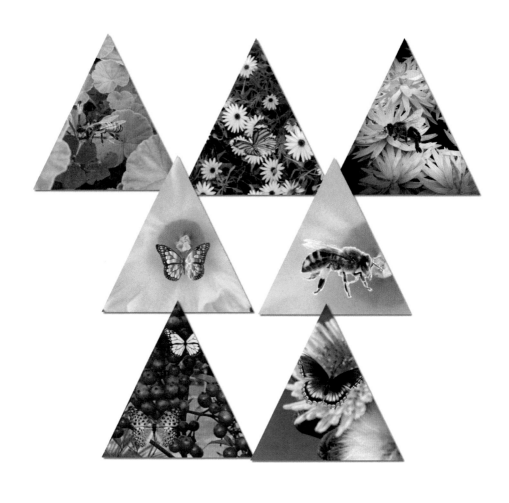

I feel grateful to your family of
insects for pollinating the plants
and teaching us teamwork.

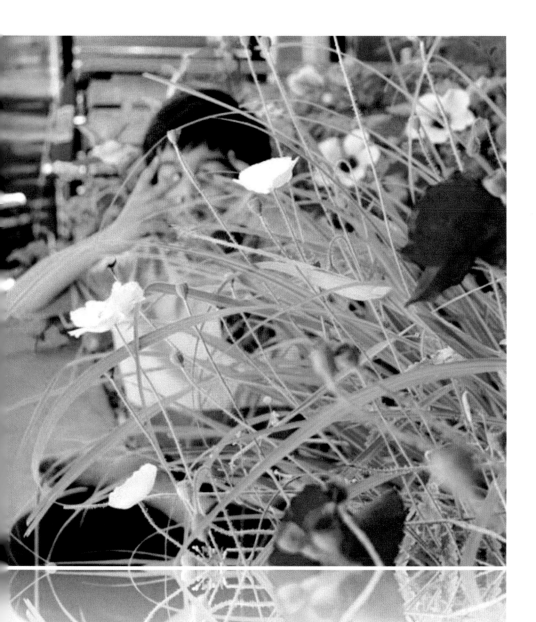

Doing Bee Breathing, I feel the vibrations of harmony with myself and nature.

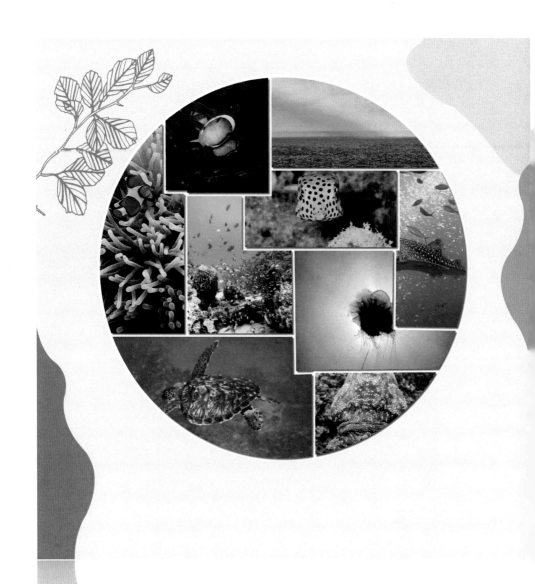

I value and respect
your oceans and
the diversity of marine life.

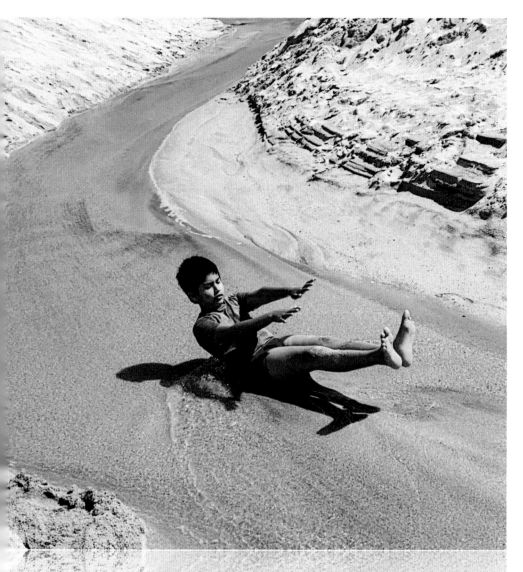

Holding myself steady in Boat Pose,
I boost my energy to stay on
course and become a champion
for saving the oceans.

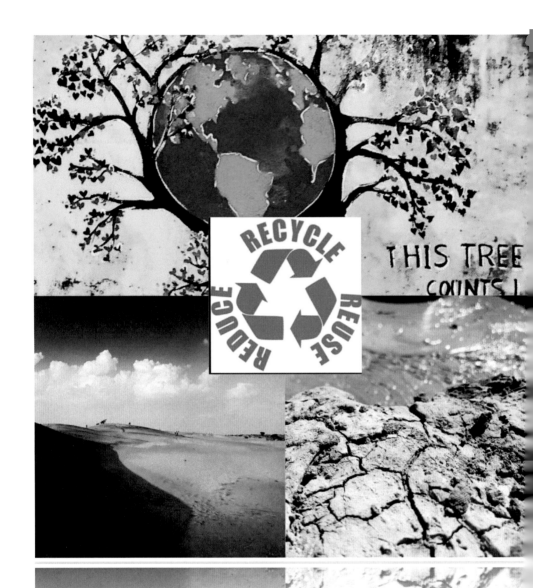

RECYCLE

REDUCE

REUSE

THIS TREE COUNTS !

I know by cutting down your trees and polluting you in many ways, we are making you uninhabitable.

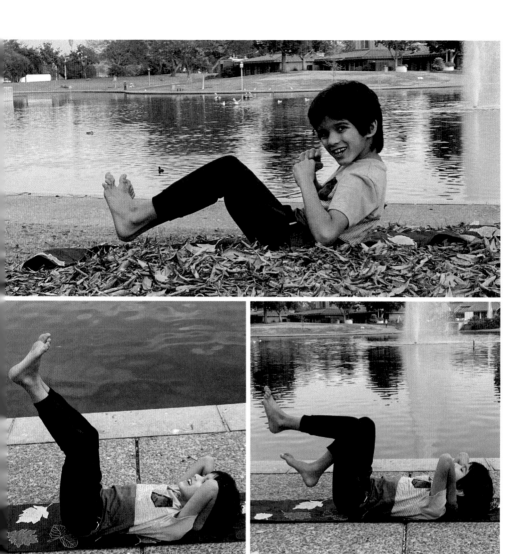

The Cycling Pose reminds me that I must support efforts to "Reduce, Reuse and Recycle" to help sustain the environment for future generations.

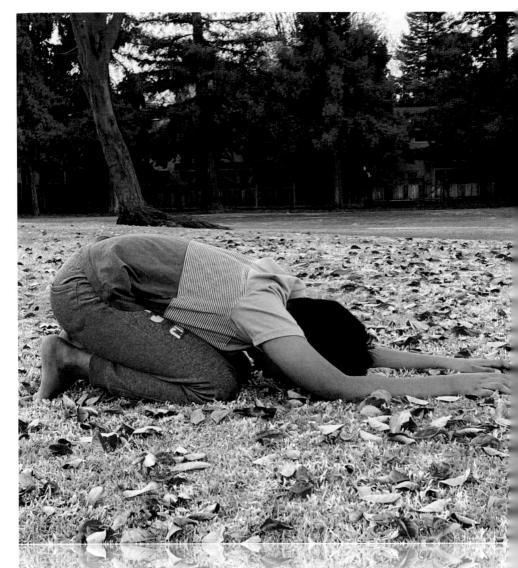

Relaxing in Child's Pose, I feel your motherly touch. Please give me the wisdom to contribute my part to care for and protect all forms of life on Earth.

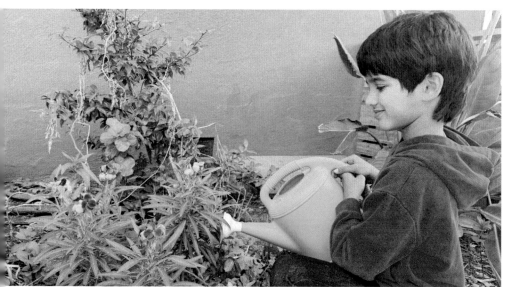

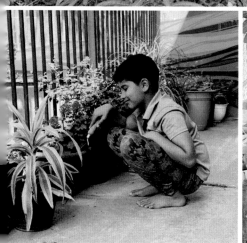
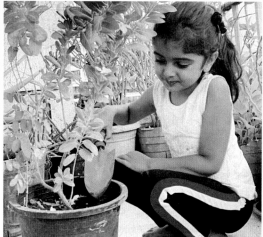

I know wishful thinking is not
enough. I can start doing my
part right now by planting
a few seeds in your fertile soil
while sitting in Squat Pose.

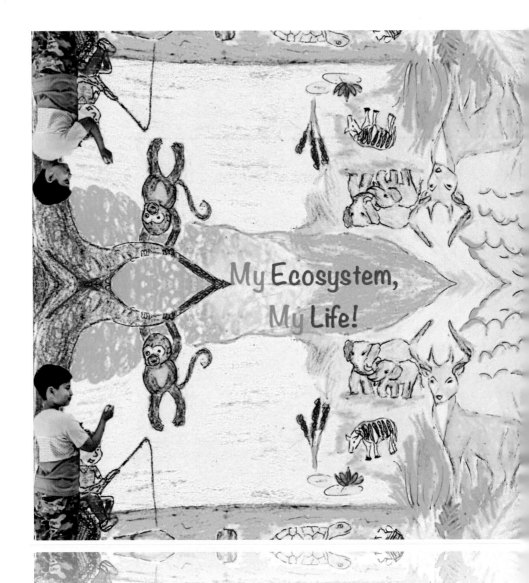

I am indebted to all of your seen and unseen, known and unknown, big, tiny, and microscopic species, who are all part of a healthy ecosystem.

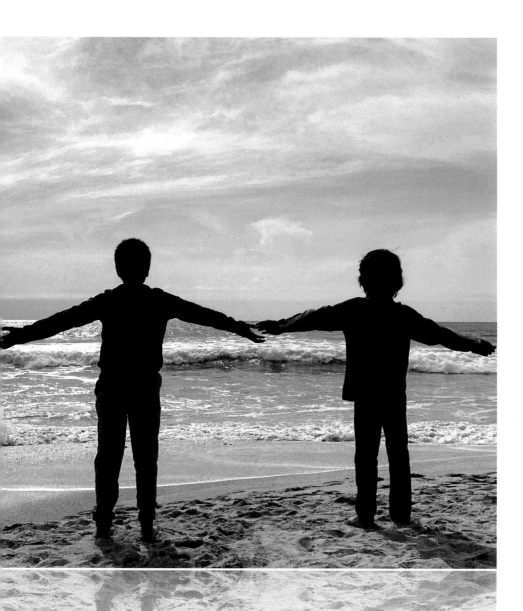

Thank you for nurturing me in every possible way and providing me with the conditions I need to live and grow.
NAMASTE EARTH!

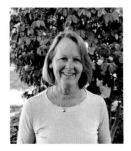

Author

Holly Love, MA is a pediatric occupational therapist, Certified YogaKids Teacher and Registered Yoga Teacher. Designing creative learning experiences for children is something Holly has done passionately for many years both professionally and with her own children.

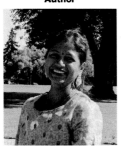

Author

Madhusmita Sahu is a Certified Yoga Instructor and an expert in the field of yoga for children. Software engineer by profession, she has a vision and passion for spreading yoga extensively and has dedicated her life to it. Madhu loves teaching, cooking, helping people, reading good books, making new friends and listening to music.

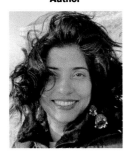

Author

Shalini Soni, the founder of Namaskar School of Yoga, is a Registered Yoga Teacher, corporate lawyer, and YouTuber. With her two awesome kids, she enjoys reading books and making videos for her YouTube channel. Shalini loves traveling, teaching, writing, public speaking and is currently available for workshops on yoga.

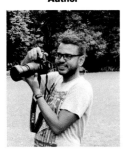

Photographer

Anand Deo is a Certified Yoga Instructor, founder of Ananda Foundation (an NGO), a YouTuber, and a true cosmopolitan. Quitting his corporate job, he has embarked on a journey of traveling, photography, and helping people realize their dreams in many ways. As a solo traveler, Anand has traveled to more than 70 countries and is still exploring the world!

Website: www.namaskarschoolofyoga.com

Youtube channel: Namaskar School of Yoga

Contact at: namaskarschoolofyoga@gmail.com

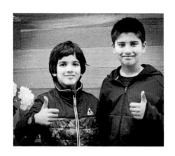

Praise for *Namaste Earth*

"I can easily imagine that Namaste Earth would have been a mainstay in my Yoga Garden classes, as well as a constant in my children's favorite childhood books. It's a lovely work of art."
-Jennifer Durand, founder of Tea & Yoga Society and creator of The Yoga Garden Game

"Namaste Earth is a beautiful tribute to nature through child-friendly yoga poses. The engaging text and bright photos are a fun way to help children practice simple poses while learning about yoga's interconnectedness with nature. Written by children's yoga teachers with years of experience, Namaste Earth is a delightful, and thoughtful picture book."
-Alicia H., Youth Librarian